Herbs versus Pharmaceuticals

Natural remedies made from herbs have been proven to be highly effective in treating and preventing a lot of health conditions, usually without the unpleasant side effects that would have occurred with the use of modern medications. They are also easy to obtain, cost effective, and less harmful to the body in the long-run.

Too much use of drugs, besides the potentially harmful side effects, can do a lot of potential damage to the organs. Among the most commonly known health hazards from overmedication is too much toxins in the blood, which can then put a strain on the liver to filter detoxify and metabolize the chemicals. Natural remedies, although often work like drugs in the body, provide one with all the healing benefits with little to no dangerous by products, which makes them a safer option for self-healing.

Despite their benefits, however, it should be noted that natural remedies are not the sole solution to all health conditions, nor are they completely danger-free either. In fact, when not use properly, herbal formulas can be just as deadly! Hence, both herbal medicines and pharmaceuticals do have their rightful place, and neither should completely replace the other. So, before you begin to stock up the kitchen cabinets with medicinal herbs, you first need to know about Dos and Don'ts of using natural remedies.

When to use natural remedies:

- **Your condition does not require a doctor's assessment and prescription medications.** Natural remedies work bests for common conditions, such as a cold, sore throat, indigestion and coughs. As a general rule, if all you need are an over-the-counter (OTC) medication and a lot of rest to feel better, you can consider substituting medication for an herbal remedy.

- **You are not sick at all.** If you are feeling fatigued or stressed out, an herbal preparation can be taken as a preventive measure to boost immunity. Unlike medications that are taken only when needed, many herbal formulas can be used daily to maintain well-being (see Chapter 3 for recipes).

- **You are in optimal health.** Only opt for herbal remedies when you are feeling under the weather if you are not suffering from a chronic condition, are not on long-term prescription medication, and have no known allergies to any herbs.

When you should NOT use natural remedies:

- **You have taken medication for your condition within the last 12-24 hours.** Herbal formulas can have deadly chemical interactions with medication. If you decide to switch to herbal remedies from your OTC, wait at least a day for the medication to clear from your system, just to be safe.

- **You have been diagnosed with a chronic condition and are taking prescription medication.** If you have a serious health condition that requires long-term medication use, consult a doctor before using any

Legal & Disclaimer

The information contained in this book is not designed to replace or take the place of any form of medicine or professional medical advice. The information in this book has been provided for educational and entertainment purposes only.

The information contained in this book has been compiled from sources deemed reliable, and it is accurate to the best of the Author's knowledge; however, the Author cannot guarantee its accuracy and validity and cannot be held liable for any errors or omissions. Changes are periodically made to this book. You must consult your doctor or get professional medical advice before using any of the suggested remedies, techniques, or information in this book.

Upon using the information contained in this book, you agree to hold harmless the Author from and against any damages, costs, and expenses, including any legal fees potentially resulting from the application of any of the information provided by this guide. This disclaimer applies to any damages or injury caused by the use and application, whether directly or indirectly, of any advice or information presented, whether for breach of contract, tort, negligence, personal injury, criminal intent, or under any other cause of action.

You agree to accept all risks of using the information presented inside this book. You need to consult a professional medical practitioner in order to ensure you are both able and healthy enough to participate in this program.

Introduction

Herbs have always been a part of our daily lives. We often use them to add flavors to the foods we make. Traces of herbal ingredients can be widely found in our toiletries, the health supplements we take for our well-being, and the medicine that treats illnesses. Despite their ubiquity, the true health and medicinal properties of herbs are at their most potent when used in their natural, unprocessed state, just the way they are found in the wilderness.

The enormous benefits to be had from incorporating more use of herbal solutions in your life cannot be overstated. You will save money from less frequent visits to the doctor or pharmacy, safe yourself from the unpleasant side effects of drugs, and reduce the amount of chemicals you come in contact with when using hygiene products. Generally, you can look forward to a pleasant and less chemically-saturated household environment, which will have an immense impact on your overall health.

Of course, to reap the rewards that nature has to offer, a foundational knowledge of herbalism is required. This guide focuses on the medicinal uses of herbs for common illnesses and overall well-being. You will learn about some of the most commonly found herbs, their uses, and how to safely prepare them for consumption or external use.

This guide is by no means an extensive resource on herbalism; the subject is too wide-encompassing to be covered in a few hundred pages, nor can it be realistically mastered over a period of weeks. It should also be said that information presented here is not meant as a substitute to professional medical advice and care. So, whenever in doubt or in cases of serious illnesses, exercise caution by seeking guidance from a qualified healthcare professional or a professional herbalist.

What you will gain here is the fundamental knowledge of herbalism, and how to start using natural remedies safely. Should you wish to deepen your knowledge of natural remedies, the final chapter offers a list of authoritative sources for further learning.

Chapter 1

Herbs at Home

Before the advent of modern medicine, people have always relied on nature for answers and remedies to ailments. The use of herbs for health care never actually loses its place; many of pharmaceuticals contain chemical compounds that derived from plant sources. Not only that, almost all the products we used on our bodies – shampoos, soaps and lotions – contain herbal ingredients and chemical components to some degree. While such modern conveniences no doubt make life easier, it also creates several potential problems to our health and the planet in the long-run. This is because most the products and drugs we are accustomed to contain more harsh chemicals that far exceed the herbal compounds.

The truth is nature's potent healing wonders – in their organic, unaltered and unprocessed form – are easily accessible. All one has to do is learn about the types of herbs available, their many uses and the necessary precautions to take.

herbal remedies or health supplements. You should not under any circumstances stop your medication without getting a green light from a doctor.

- **Your condition does not improve after 5-7 days.** If you have been self-medicating with herbal remedies and getting enough rest, but feeling no signs of recovering, it is time to cease whatever you are taking and see a doctor.

9 Rules for Safe Self-Healing

It should be reminded that although natural remedies are generally safe, herbs still work like drugs in the body in that they do cause chemical reactions. Hence, when considering self-medication with homemade herbal substances, always follow these safety precautions.

1. **Be absolutely certain of the remedy you plan on using.** Make sure you got the right herb, at the right dosage, prepared with the right method, and it is the remedy for your condition. There should be no room for guest work when using an herbal formula.

2. **Do not self-medicate if your condition is critical.** Never use homemade remedies for severe conditions that require emergency medical attention. Likewise, if symptoms of you condition persist – high fever that would not subside, coughing that gets worse or pain does not go away – seek the attention of a healthcare professional.

3. **Do not assume an herbal preparation is safe.** Homemade natural remedies do not necessarily have to be made with fresh herbs; some herbs can be purchased in other forms such as powder, essential oils or teabags. Herb-based products are normally not regulated by the Food and Drug Administration (FDA) for safety or efficacy. If you need to purchase an herbal preparation to be used as an ingredient in your home remedy, search the label for a seal of approval from the USP (United States Pharmacopeia), or CL (Consumer-Lab.com). This would indicate that it has been approved by certified academic laboratories. If you do not see any, do a quick research about the brand before buying.

4. **Sample before using.** It is not wise to use an herbal remedy that you are unfamiliar with for the first time when you are ill. The best time to ensure that a substance is safe for you is to try it out when you are in perfect health. After all, almost all herbs are safe to be consumed on a daily basis as health tonics. So, go lower than the recommended dosage and give it a try. Even if you are only using a formula externally, such as homemade lotions or scrubs, do a patch test by applying a small amount to your skin first. Sampling a formula before you commit to using it is a good way to check for rare side effects and allergic reactions.

5. **Observe yourself.** Much of successful self-healing has to do with knowing your own body. Whether you are ill or not, always pay attention to physiological changes to your body and health when using natural substances. Be mindful of the time of usage, dosage

and resulting effects, and then tweak your usage to suit your needs. For instance, if you choose to take a cup of ginger after dinner for a week to aid digestion, watch out for how the body responds. You may notice you feel less gassy than you normally do after a heavy meal, so perhaps you would like to make it an after-meal habit. You should also observe for allergic reactions and stop the use of a certain herb immediately is you find out you are allergic to it.

6. **Do not overdo it.** More is not necessarily better, and could be dangerous. Always adhere to recommended dosages, and when uncertain, it is better to err on the side of caution by sticking to a low dosage.

7. **Never mix meds and herbs.** The mixture of medications and herbal concoctions make a lethal cocktail that should not be taken lightly! <u>Never ever use herbal remedies alongside prescription of OTC medications.</u> Some herbs – even in small and diluted quantities – can interact with certain medications, including those for hypertension, diabetes and blood thinners. If you have to be on medication, be sure to have open discussion with a physician about considering herbal alternatives.

8. **Whenever in doubt, do not proceed.** Unless you receive advice from a qualified herbalist or holistic healing practitioner, it is better not to attempt using any natural remedies that involve using herbs you are unfamiliar with. This rule especially applies using to rare and potent herbs to treat a health condition.

9. **Exercise extra precaution with pregnant women and children.** Women who are pregnant or nursing should consult a qualified healthcare practitioner before consuming any herbal concoctions. Children under the age of 12 should not use herbal remedies.

Chapter 2

Essential Herbs

There are hundreds and thousands of useful herbs out there that it would take a lifetime of dedicated learning to know about all of them. Even so, you only need a foundational knowledge of some of the most common herbs to start using and benefit from natural remedies. The list presented here is a dozen common herbs that should have a place in your kitchen pantry. They are easy to identify, obtain and prepared for safe usage. Although focus will be given to their medicinal use, these herbs can also be used as cooking ingredients to add flavors and health benefits to your daily meals.

Ginger

In traditional eastern medicine, ginger is hailed as the miracle herb since ancient times, and there are plenty of scientific evidence to back that claim. A powerful antioxidant, ginger stops the production of free radicals and blocks out the effect of serotonin, a chemical produced by the brain and stomach that causes you to feel nauseated. Ginger also helps regulate blood flow and lower blood pressure. It has anti-inflammatory properties, making it effective in reducing joint and muscle pain. When used as a food ingredient or taken as tea after meal, ginger stimulates the body to release proper enzymes that aid digestion and nutrient absorption, while also easing stomach gas and bloating. There are even a few studies suggesting that long-term regular ginger intake can lower the risk of ovarian cancer in women.

Uses:
- Avert nausea caused by upset stomach, indigestion, motion sickness or cancer treatment
- Relieve gas and bloating after a heavy meal
- Pain relief from muscle soreness, arthritis, and menstrual cramps
- Relief from upper respiratory tract infections, coughs and bronchitis
- Relief from allergy symptoms
- Provide heat and energy on during cold weather

Peppermint

With archeological evidence placing its usage as far back as 10,000 years ago, peppermint is often regarded as the world's oldest medicine. Its place in the field of natural cures is hardly surprising; peppermint is rich in manganese, Vitamin A and C. To top it off, it is known for being pleasant to the taste buds, it is among the easiest herbs to grow, and its usage carries minimal risk. Peppermint is commonly used to sooth stomach discomforts, relieving indigestion and vomiting. Crushed leaves or oils can be applied to skin to soothe muscle soreness.

Uses:

- Relief from upset stomach, indigestion and flatulence
- Inhibit bacterial growth, especially in the digestive tract
- Treats mild food poisoning
- Treat fevers
- Relieve sinus congestion
- Reduce irritable bowel syndrome
- Treats spastic colon

Chamomile

The medicinal powers of chamomile are found in the delicate, apple-scented white blossoms. Chamomile is a natural antihistamine, which make it effective in treating nervous stress and inflammations. Its reputation as a medicinal plant comes from its rich anti-inflammatory, anti-bacterial, muscle relaxant, antispasmodic, anti-allergenic and sedative properties. There is no better way to unwind after a stressful day than with a cup of chamomile tea!

Uses:

- Reduces anxiety and nervous stress
- Relieves stomach disorders, infections and skin inflammation
- Induces relaxation
- Promote restful sleep
- Relief from allergic symptoms

Rosemary

Traditionally used to sharpen concentration and memory, Rosemary may just be the herbal answer to caffeinated beverages for a jolt of alertness. As a stimulant, rosemary promotes brain health by bringing more oxygen to the brain. Rosemary is a favorite ingredient in many Mediterranean dishes for several reasons; besides adding aroma and flavor to meat, it has cancer fighting properties. Frying, broiling, or grilling meats at high temperatures creates potent carcinogens implicated in several cancers. The two powerful antioxidants found in rosemary, carnosol and rosemarinic acid, are known to destroy carcinogens, thus lowering the risk of cancerous tumors forming in the body. Furthermore, a pot of rosemary is not only a nice ornamental plant, but also gives off a pleasant aroma and keeps mosquitoes away.

Uses:
- Stimulates digestive, circulatory and nervous systems to promotes cleansing of the body
- A rich source of antioxidant that helps boost the immune system
- Improves blood circulation
- Prevents brain aging
- Enhance memory and concentration
- Prolonged regular consumption is said to prevent cancerous tumors

Holy Basil

Several animal studies have shown that holy basil – a special variety of the basil plant – is effective in handling stress by regulating stress hormones released by the adrenal glands that a trigger fight-or-flight response, such as adrenalin and corticosterone. In moderate amounts, stress hormones boost mental clarity, alertness and memory, which come in handy in helping us cope with a distressing situation. In other words, as an adaptogen, holy basil enhances the body's natural response to physical and emotional stress. Rather than having a sedative effect and altering mood, holy basil helps the body function optimally during times of stress.

Uses:
- Reduce stress-related physiological symptoms, such as digestive problems and headache
- Long-term use is said to improve memory and reduce risk of age-related mental disorders
- Lowers risk of anxiety disorders and depression
- Enhance mental clarity

Lavender

Long favored for its sweet and soothing perfume, lavender is an herb where its medicinal properties can be experience just by smelling it. The herb's scent is known to clam and relax the mind as a mild antidepressant. In fact, lavender is a versatile herb that can be consumed or used externally. Even its fresh flowers can be added to salads, cookies and bread in small doses for added taste.

Uses:
- Calms the nervous systems
- Alleviate mental and emotional stress
- Relief from insomnia and promotes restful sleep
- Used externally as an antiseptic to treat sunburn and acne
- Eases pain when applied externally to cuts and bruises

Rose

Commonly recognized for its beauty and fragrance, rose is actually one of the most potent herbal remedies that is beneficial to the body inside and out. Rose petals are high in fiber, antioxidants and antibacterial compounds, and can be used in various preparations, from drinkable tonics to massage oils.

Uses:
- Alleviate pre-menstrual symptoms (PMS)
- Soothe allergy and asthma symptoms
- Alleviate moodiness, anxiety and depression
- Relief from headaches cause by stress
- Aid digestion and detoxification
- Combat hemorrhoids
- Improves metabolism and aid weight loss
- Moisturize and soften skin
- Balances oily skin
- Treats irritation on sensitive skin
- Treats acne
- Has anti-aging properties on skin

Cinnamon

Made from the inner bark of the cinnamomum tree, cinnamon is commonly used as a spice for food and pastry for its distinct aroma and flavor. Cinnamon is packed with antioxidants, anti-inflammatory, anti-fungal and antibacterial properties, which are scientifically proven to immensely beneficial to the immune system. Most of cinnamon's benefits are experienced with prolonged regular moderate consumption, which can lead to lower risks of many illnesses like diabetes, heart diseases and cancer. However, large amount of the spice can be too potent and dangerous. So, stick to the safe recommended dosage (see Chapter 3 for recipes).

Uses:
- Improve some key risk factors for heart disease, including cholesterol, triglycerides and blood pressure
- Increase sensitivity to the hormone insulin and significantly reducing the risks of metabolic syndrome and type 2 diabetes
- Reduce fasting blood sugar levels up to 10-29%, which is a potent anti-diabetic effect
- Reduce bacterial infections
- Help fight tooth decay and bad breath

Thyme

With its delicate stems and tiny leaves, thyme is another culinary staple in the Mediterranean known for its distinctive taste. Its medicinal properties are nothing short of impressive. Thyme is just as potent in its essential oil preparation as it would when used fresh; the active principle in thyme, thymol, is a strong antiseptic. The herb is also rich in Vitamins A and C, which makes it effective as an immunity booster, especially when the weather is cold. Plus, it's also a good source of copper, fiber, iron and manganese.

Uses:
- Relief from indigestion and flatulence
- Alleviate coughs, sore throat and symptoms of acute bronchitis
- Repels insects and pests (when used in oil form)

- Natural skin deodorant
- Natural fungal disinfectant

Aloe Vera

Take a walk down the skincare and hygiene products isle at the supermarket and you will find numerous products that boast the benefits of aloe vera. The aloe plant easily identified by its thick pointy leaves that store water. The source of its medicinal powers is the slimy, water-filled tissue within the leaves, often called the gel. The aloe vera gel contains many bioactive compounds including vitamins, minerals, amino acids and antioxidants that are highly valued within the food, pharmaceutical and cosmetic industry. Of course, nothing can be compared to using an herb fresh and unprocessed. The gel can be used to make juices and desserts, but are more commonly used externally as topical applications to the skin for its soothing antibacterial properties.

Uses:
- Accelerate the healing of sunburns
- Used as mouthwash to reduce dental plaque buildup and tooth decay
- Accelerate the healing of mouth ulcers
- As laxative to treat constipation
- Improve skin elasticity and prevent wrinkles

Garlic

In folklores and superstitions, garlic is known to protect oneself from vampire attacks. In truth, garlic is a wondrous herb that can protect our organs from many harmful diseases. Garlic contains more than 70 active phytochemicals that are responsible for combating hypertension, prevent stroke, improve cholesterol levels, and clear arterial blockages. It is also known to be rich in Vitamin C, Vitamin B6, manganese, and trace amounts of various other nutrients like calcium, copper, potassium, iron and phosphorus. Perhaps the biggest benefit to be had from garlic, as vouched for by the scientific and medical field, is that regular consumption is shown to lower rates of many types of cancers. What's more, garlic is one of the easiest herbs to be included in your regular diet.

Uses:
- Boost immune system
- Lower blood pressure
- Improve cholesterol levels
- Improve overall cardiovascular health
- Lower risks of cancer

Parsley

Often used as a garnish to add a little color to a dish, parsley is more than meets the eye. The decorative green herb has one of the highest levels of chlorophyll, which can help boost immunity, lower inflammation and clear toxins form the body. Additionally, parsley contains alpha-linolenic acid, the omega-3 fatty acid that is beneficial to the heart. It is also rich in many vitamins, including Vitamin C, B 12, K and A.

Uses:
- Strengthen immune and nervous system

- Promote healthy kidney function by helping to flush out excess fluids from the body (Precaution: parsley contains oxalates, which can cause problems for those with existing kidney and gall bladder problems)
- Relief from arthritic joint pains
- Relaxes stiff muscles and encourages digestion
- Reduce hair loss when essential oil is massaged onto the scalp
- Prolonged regular use helps with controlling blood pressure and prevention of cardiovascular diseases

Chapter 3

Healing at Home

Why swallow pills that will leave you feeling drugged up when a solution can easily be found in your kitchen? These natural remedy recipe templates involve the common herbs detailed in Chapter 2, and ingredients that can be easily found at the grocer. Not only will these herbal preparations save you a trip to the pharmacy when you are sick, most of them can be taken daily for their health benefits, unless mentioned otherwise.

Obtaining the Herbs You Need

Rightfully, herbs should be obtained fresh from their natural habitat in the wild. Realistically though, unless you live by the countryside, this is not a feasible method for many people. Moreover, foraging for wild plants is a field of expertise on its own that requires extensive studying. Fortunately, all the herbs used for these recipes can be easily obtained at a grocer.

Herbs come in different preparations. For example, you can buy a fresh ginger root, ginger essential oil, ginger powder, ready-made ginger teabags or even ginger capsules. All forms of preparations have their usage, although caution should be exercised to know which forms are edible and which are only meant for external use.

Store-bought preparations do not necessarily take away from you reaping the natural benefits of the herbs. There may be times when you need certain formulas, such essential oils, powder forms and exotic tea blends, that would be highly impractical to make it yourself at home. However, you do need to be an informed consumer when shopping for herbal products. When buying fresh or dried herbs, be sure to get them from reputable sources, ideally organic. The same goes for herbal products; you should buy from reputable brands and makers that can vouch for the authenticity and quality of their products. You do not want to risk poisoning and other potential health hazards from herbs that are intended for healing!

For the purpose of this guide, stay away from any herbal products that come in tablet form or marketed as health supplements. Such products fall in the category of pharmaceuticals, and often contain insolated components and extracts from herbs that can be too concentrated and strong. They should only be taken with the guidance of a healthcare professional. The recipes here use herbs and herbal products that do not isolate, alter or process the plants' chemical components.

Lastly, you can also get herbs by learning to grow your own at home (see Chapter 5).

Some Herbs a Day, Keeps Stress at Bay

Many of the common health problems – colds, flu, sore throat, indigestion, headache and sleeplessness – have their root cause in stress. Alas, stress is an inevitable part of life. No matter how good we become at handling and managing stress, it occasionally gets the better of us. Stress is responsible for making you feel emotionally and physically tense, making your digestive system go awry, keeping you from getting the much needed restful sleep at night, and thus compromising your immune system and overall well-being.

The beauty of natural remedies is that they do not always have to be used only when you are ill. In fact, as you should have learned by now, the benefits of many herbs in combating diseases are experienced from prolonged regular use. Moreover, herbalism is a form of holistic healing where optimal health is attained by nourishing the whole person – body, mind, emotions and spirit. So, it only makes sense to incorporate more herbs into your daily life for regular health maintenance.

The following recipes are meant as templates to give you the simplest ways to prepare and consume more herbs on a daily basis, not just as treatment for illness. Feel free to modify, experiment and adapt them to suit your individual needs.

Herbal Teas

Nothing soothes the mind and heals the body like a cup of warm tea! Herbal teas are the most convenient and safe of natural remedies. All you need is hot water and an herb of your choice, fresh or dried. Raw honey and lemon can be added for taste if desired. Furthermore, herbal teas can serve as a basis to make other remedies by adding in other ingredients. Drink a cup of herbal tea at the first sign of a cold, for relief of symptoms, after a heavy meal, or anytime of the day when you need to unwind from the events of a hectic day.

While the simple recipe given here are meant for brewing tea with a single herb, as you continue building on your knowledge of herbalism, you may try making unique tea blends by mixing two or more herbs.

Dosage: 2-4 cups a day, every 3-4 hours or whenever needed. While beneficial to your health, teas can be dehydrating. So, be sure to balance your daily dose of herbal teas with adequate water intake. To avoid dehydration, drink 2 cups of water for every cup of tea.

Ingredients: leaves of peppermint, thyme, holy basil, parsley or rosemary; lavender or chamomile flowers; rose petals; ginger slices; cinnamon chips (pick one that suits your needs. See Chapter 2 for medicinal properties of each herb)

Directions:
1. If using fresh herbs, wash thoroughly and crush them properly.
2. Put a teaspoon of dried, or a small handful of crushed fresh herb of your choice into a cup or teapot. You may adjust this quantity to suit your personal preference for milder or stronger taste, just be careful not to overdo it.

3. Pour boiled hot water over the herbs, close a lid over, and leave to steep for 5-10 minutes.
4. Strain tea into another cup.
5. Add a slice of lemon or raw honey for taste if desired (optional).
6. Enjoy!

Precaution: Do not reuse herbs! Once you finished brewing a cup of tea, throw the used herbs away. A second cup of tea brewed from used herbs loses flavor and strength.

Healing Smoothies

Drinking smoothies is a great way to make up for the lack of fruits and vegetables in your diet. Plus, making them is easy; just assemble the ingredients in a blender, blend together and enjoy. A well-made cup of smoothie is packed with all the nutritional goodness of its fruits and vegetables ingredients, why not add some herbs to your smoothie recipes? This will give your wholesome beverages some extra flavor and added health benefits.

There are plenty of smoothie recipes out there, but the best ones are those of your own creation. The following is a template for smoothie recipes, which you can experiment with and adapt to suit your taste buds' content:

- 0.5-2 servings* of a fruits or vegetables (you can use 1-3 different types of fruits and vegetables)
- 1-2 cups of cold water or chilled herbal tea
- 1-3 teaspoons of additives (raw honey, syrup or any natural flavoring
- 1 handful of herb

Directions:
1. Thoroughly washed fruits and vegetables, and have them properly chopped up for easy blending.
2. Put all ingredients in the blender, fruits first.
3. Blend to the desired consistency.

* A serving is roughly measured by what fits into the palm of your hand. For example, a banana, an apple or a cup of berries are counted as one serving.

Making delicious smoothies may require some trial-and-error. Once you found the right combination, note down the recipe, and share your personalized beverage with loved ones! To take some guesswork out of the process, here are some suggested combinations for six herbs that would make great additions to smoothies and how they can be added to the blend:

Ginger
Use: fresh root or a pinch of shredded dried ginger
Suggested combinations: apple, banana, orange, lemon, pear, pumpkin, nut milk, figs, dates, tropical fruits, carrot, chocolate, vegetable juices, leafy greens, green tea

Cinnamon
Use: ground cinnamon or whole sticks
Suggested combinations: apple, pear, banana, coconut, nut milk, dates, pumpkin, coffee, tea, vanilla, chocolate

Holy Basil (or any variety of basil)
Use: add a pinch of fresh leaves into the blender

Suggested combinations: honey melon, red berries, citrus fruit, pineapple, leafy greens, blueberry

Lavender
Use: fresh or dried flowers; use sparingly because lavender is a potent herb
Suggested combinations: red berries, vanilla, white tea, chocolate, raw honey, white chocolate, blueberry, pear, orange

Peppermint
Use: fresh leaves
Suggested combinations: Lime, grapefruit, lemon, chocolate, melon, red berries, blueberry, blackberry, cucumber

Rose
Use: fresh petals
Suggested combinations: oolong tea, green tea, citrus fruit, nut milk, coffee, apple, pear, raw honey

Homemade Aloe Vera Juice

A glass of aloe vera juice is a refreshing treat on a hot day. It detoxifies the body and strengthens the immune system, and makes an excellent remedy to relieve constipation.

Unlike other herbs where their uses are very straight forward, there is a method to preparing aloe vera that requires extra care. Aloe vera has a lot of medicinal benefits to the body, but it is also has a toxic part of the leaf that needs to be removed safely and properly before you can use the gel. Otherwise, it could lead to diarrhea and stomach cramps. When taking aloe vera gel internally, do not exceed 1-2 teaspoons of a day and no more than five days a week. Exceeding this amount may result in serious side effects.

To prepare aloe vera gel:
1. Break off a large ripe leaf and wash it under running water to clean away mud and dirt.
2. Dry it with an absorbent cloth and let the rind dry completely.
3. With a knife or kitchen scissors, cut off the edges to remove the thorny part. This will make opening the leaf easier.
4. With a sharp knife, peel the rind on one side and the yellow layer just beneath the rind. Discard.
5. Once all the rind and yellow gel beneath it have been removed, you should be left with only clear aloe vera gel.
6. Scoop out the gel with a spoon. Be careful not to scrape the yellowish layer and rind at the bottom; your extracted gel should be clear, without any of the yellowish or greenish stuff.

By following these steps, you should be able to get approximately 2 tablespoons of gel from one leaf. Use immediately, when the gel is freshly extracted. Remember you only need 1-2 teaspoons for one serving, so put the remaining unused gel in an airtight jar and refrigerate it. Do not keep or use the gel that is more than three days-old or when it changes to a yellowish color, it means the gel has oxidized.

To make the juice:
- 2 tsp aloe vera gel

- 1 cup of water, or any vegetable or fruit juice, preferably freshly squeezed
- Raw honey as sweetener

Gather materials in a blender, blend and serve immediately.

Garlic to the Rescue

Because of its many different ways of preparation and medicinal potency, the uses for garlic deserve special attention. Garlic is not a popular herb to be taken fresh because of its pungent odor, and eating excessive amounts does cause bad breath, body odor, indigestion, and mouth irritation. Yet, garlic works best as a remedy when eaten raw, as over-cooking may destroy its medicinal properties.

Garlic also thins the blood, lowers glucose levels and increases insulin. So, if you are on any blood thinners or drugs that lower blood sugar, avoid taking garlic. Because garlic increases the risk of bleeding, pregnant women should not use it as a remedy.

If you are feeling under the weather, especially from a cold, the following three garlic recipes may be all you need to feel better. Like most natural remedies, you can also take these garlic preparations to boost immunity and prevent diseases. If you are recovering from a cold, you may take any of these garlic remedies three times a day, at four hours intervals. Do not exceed three helpings, and be sure to drink plenty of water.

Raw Garlic

Eating fresh garlic cloves may not be the most pleasant thing to do, but it is the quickest and most effective cold remedy. Well, you do not have to eat; simply crush one garlic cove and suck it as a lozenge for 15 minutes. Repeat every 4 hours.

Garlic Toast

1. Mince 1-2 garlic cloves, and let it sit for 15 minutes. This is to allow the enzymes to activate.
2. Meanwhile, make toast and spread butter on it (you can use margarine or raw honey instead).
3. Sprinkle the minced garlic on the toast and eat it.
4. Eat regularly to prevent cold, ideally as breakfast.

Garlic Soup

1. Pour 8 cups vegetable or chicken broth into a large soup pot.
2. Add and stir in 1.5 tablespoons olive oil, 1 whole head of peeled and chopped garlic cloves, half a teaspoon dried thyme, and a pinch of dried sage.
3. Bring to a boil, reduce heat and let it simmer for 30 minutes.
4. Remove from heat and strain.
5. You may add salt for taste.
6. Drink this soup 3 times a day when recovering from a cold.

If you are concerned over bad breath after eating garlic, a simple solution is to chew a fresh sprig of parsley. The chlorophyll in the green herb acts as a breath freshener.

Chapter 4

Health and Beauty

Herbal formulas form the basis for many cosmetic and hygiene products we use every day. While you may get the familiar scent of your favorite herbs whenever you use those products, you are also exposing your skin to absorbing plenty of harsh chemicals. Furthermore, those chemicals in bath and beauty products get washed off and into the water, contributing to environmental pollution.

It may not be very realistic or practical to switch entirely to natural, homemade hygiene products, but you can always substitute a few items in the bathroom cabinet for stuff from made in your kitchen. By opting for the natural, chemical-free alternative – even on occasion – you are playing a part in saving the planet and yourself from harmful chemicals.

The main ingredient commonly used in natural hygiene products are essential oils from strong scented flowery herbs like lavender and rose. You will need a substance for the base, such as cocoa butter, nut oils or water, to which you will add the herbal ingredients into. You can also benefit from herbs just by adding them to your bath water. By all means, you can try out these herbal recipes that will heal you on the outside.

Rosewater for Rosy Skin

Rose petals contain antioxidants and antibacterial compounds that will soothe the skin, providing relief from excessive irritation and itching. Because of its astringent properties, rose is also beneficial in deep cleansing and toning the skin, while also fight signs of skin aging when used regularly. The flower petals also contain an antiseptic compound known as phenyl ethanol, making it effective against bacteria that cause acne. Best of all, rose works for all types of skin; it is gentle on sensitive skin, balances moisture on oily skin and returns suppleness to dry skin. It may just be the only skincare product that you will ever need!

To make rose a part of your skincare regime, you need to make rosewater. There are three of the simplest methods to making rosewater, all of which will allow you to benefit from the properties of the flower just the same. Whichever method you choose, always use distilled water. Tap water often contains bacteria. If distilled water is not available, boil filtered water and leave it to cool to room temperature.

To make rosewater with essential oil:
- 12 drop of pure rose essential oil (fragrance oil will give the rose scent and none of the medicinal benefits)
- 2 teaspoons of vodka
- 1 cup of distilled water
- Glass jar (avoid metal or plastic)

Directions:

1. Fill the jar with water.
2. Dilute 12 drops of rose essential oil with vodka on a dish. Otherwise, the oil will float and not mix with the water.
3. Add essential oil to water, close the jar tightly and shake to mix it.
4. The advantage of using this method is that your rosewater will have a longer shelf life of up to a year.

To make rosewater with fresh rose petals:

- 1 cup of rose petals (about 2 big roses)
- 2 cups of distilled water
- 1 teaspoon vodka (optional)
- Glass jar

Directions:

1. Pull the petals off, wash and rinse.
2. Evenly distribute the petals on a saucepan and pour water over them. Make sure the water level does not go too far past the petals, or else you will end up with diluted rosewater. A teaspoon of vodka may be added as preservative to make the rosewater last longer.
3. Cover the pot and turn on the stove at low heat. Do not let the water boil or reach a simmer; the heat will ruin the medicinal properties of the petals.
4. Heat for 20 minutes. The petals will then lose some color while the water will take on a reddish hue.
5. Place a strainer over the jar and pour the rosewater into it.

6. Store rosewater in the refrigerator. Rosewater made with this method would last for a week. If vodka was added, it will last up to 2 weeks.

To make rosewater with dried rose petals:
- 1/4 cup of dried rose petals
- 1.25 cup of hot distilled water
- 2 glass jars

Directions:
- Put dried rose petals into one of the jars.
- Pour hot (but not boiling) water over the petals.
- Cover the jar and let it cool.
- Once cooled, put a strainer over the empty jar and pour the rosewater into it.
- Store rosewater in the refrigerator. This method is faster than using fresh petals and cheaper than buying essential oils. However, the rosewater must be used within a week or it will expire.

To incorporate rosewater into your skincare regime, apply it to face and neck after cleansing your skin. You may put rosewater in a misting bottle and use as a spray on your skin, as deodorant, to add fragrance to linen or as room air freshener.

Natural Acne Treatment

A lot of acne topical medications contain harsh chemicals that may leave you with dry and cracking skin once the pimples are gone. This natural treatment makes use of the potent antibacterial properties of rose. It not only gets rid of acne, but also leaves your skin nourished.

Ingredients:
- Rosewater (room temperature and cold)
- 1/4-1/2 cup of fenugreek seeds

Directions:
1. Soak fenugreek seeds overnight in water.
2. Make a fine paste with the seeds by adding rosewater.
3. Apply to face as a mask and leave for 20 minutes.
4. Rinse with cold rosewater.

Calm Skin with Chamomile

Chamomile calms the nerves from the inside and also soothes the skin from the outside. To treat skin inflammation and rashes that resulted from allergic reaction, weed poisoning or other medical conditions, make an infusion of 1 teaspoon chamomile flowers per cup of hot water. Steep until cool, and apply to skin using a cool compress or use as skin wash.

Skin Soothing Chamomile-Lavender Body Cream

This sweet-smelling body cream will come in handy to soothe skin from sunburn, moisturize dryness and keep skin nourished as a night cream. It may take extra time to make, but the final product will be well worth your patience.

Ingredients
- 1/3 cup of dried chamomile flowers
- Olive oil

- 1/2 cup of cocoa butter
- 1/2 cup of coconut oil
- 1 teaspoon of pure lavender essential oil

Directions:
1. Put dried chamomile flowers into a clean and dry glass jar. Add just enough olive oil to fully immerse all the flowers.
2. Cover the jar with an unused coffee filter, securing it with a rubber band.
3. Place the jar by a sunny window to let the oil infuse for about 10 days.
4. Strain out and dispose the plant material into a glass bottle. If there is left over, store it in a cool place for future use. It should last for a year.
5. Melt cocoa butter and coconut oil into 1 cup of the chamomile infused oil.
6. Remove from heat and pour into a stainless steel bowl. Put the mixture in the freezer to begin cooling.
7. Every 5-10 minutes, take the bowl out from the freezer and whip with an electric mixer, first slowly and gradually increasing the speed each time.
8. Once the mixture reaches a creamy consistency, add 1 teaspoon of lavender essential oil and mix.
9. Spoon the cream into glass containers with air-tight lids, and store in a cool place. Your body cream is ready for use!

Homemade Insect Repellant

Mosquitoes and bugs are not only a nuisance when you spend time outdoors, they may carry diseases such as dengue fever or malaria, and their bite could be venomous. To protect yourself, you can make a homemade repellant:

Ingredients:
- 2 tablespoons of either olive, jojoba or almond oil (known as carrier oils)
- 10 drops of essential oil with insect repelling properties (thyme, rosemary, peppermint, cinnamon, citronella, lemon, tea tree or eucalyptus)

Directions:
1. Mix the carrier oil with essential oils of your choice thoroughly.
2. Apply to areas of expose skin or clothing before heading outdoors. Alternatively, you can put the repellent in a misting bottle and spray it on as needed.
3. If you need to make more, add 5 drops essential oil for every tablespoon of carrier oil. You may experiment with mixing essential oils to create an insect repellent that also smells nice.

Make Bruises Go Away

You know those unsightly black-and-blue marks you get when you bumped into something? You can speed up their disappearance with a simple treatment. Just crush a handful of parley (or as much as you need) with mortar and pestle, then applied repeatedly to a bruise.

Chapter 5

Creating Your Herb Garden

As you use more herbs and your knowledge of herbalism expands, you will want to have a convenient supply of herbs. What better way to get fresh herbs than from your own garden? Herbs are generally easy to grow and care for, whether in a garden or in a pot by a sunny windowsill indoors. However, growing herbs, much like using them, does has its learning curves.

What Are You Growing?

Before you indulge your green thumb, you have to first decide what you want to grow. It is best to start with one or two herbs that you use regularly, and gradually expand your garden as you from there. Many leafy and flowery herbs, including those introduced in Chapter 2, can be purchased in a pot from supermarkets or gardening centers. You can also find seeds of common herbs that you can germinate and grow on your own.

Annual, Biennial or Perennial?

Just because you are growing your own herbs, it does not mean you will have a constant supply of herbs at your disposal. When starting your garden, it is worth knowing whether your chosen herb is annual, biennial or perennial:

Annuals – Herbs that fall into this category are plants that go through the entire life cycle from seed to flower to seed within a single growing season. Basically, all roots, stems and leaves of the plant die annually. Only the dormant seeds will sprout the next generation.

Biennials – Plants of this category complete their life cycle in two years. The first season of growth results in small flowers and leaves, close to the soil surface. The second season of growth boasts long stems. Flowering and see formation would occur, followed by the entire plant's death.

Perennials – Plants that grow for many seasons. Generally, such plants go into dormancy at some point of the year, with the top portion dying off each winter and re-growing the following spring from the same root system.

Annual and biennial herbs are fast growing and may need sowing at intervals throughout spring and summer, if you want to have a continuous fresh supply. Examples of such herbs include basil, coriander, parsley, dill, chamomile and lemongrass. On the other hand, perennial herbs are slower growing and will require a more permanent home. Herbs that fall into this category include mint, thyme, rosemary, sage, oregano, lemon balm and chives There are also plants that can behave as an annual or perennial, depending on the geographic and climate of the growing condition. Knowing how a plant behaves is essential, as it will determine how you have to care for them.

Basic Herbal Plant Care

The ideal growing condition for your herbs is a sunny, sheltered location, with well-drained and pH neutral soil. This applies whether the plants are growing in an outdoor garden or in containers and pots indoors. Water the plants at the base of the plant when the soil begins to feel dry, at least once per week. However, there are certain plants that do not tolerate direct sunlight and require less or more frequent watering. So, if you do not have experience in growing herbs, talk to the keepers the gardening centers or store when purchasing the plants. Ask them for proper caring tips and instructions.

Be sure to keep the surrounding soil clean and pull weeds that appear near the plant, so that they will not steal the nutrients from the soil. If growing outdoors, bring them in or under a shelter before the first frost.

Harvesting

Once the plants are ready for harvesting, pick the leaves or flowers with your fingers, or for a cleaner harvest, snip them with kitchen shears. Pick the mature leaves and flowers at the top, and do not pick the stems bare; you want to allow the plants to re-grow.

Using and Storing the Herbs

It is best to harvest the herbs at the time you want to use them to ensure freshness. Be sure to wash them thoroughly to remove bugs, dirt and soil. If you need to store herbs for later use, you can either dry them or freeze them. As always, you need to wash them properly and gently remove excess water by patting with a paper towel.

- **To dry herbs:** Cut the stems at soil level, tie a bunch together at the bottom of the stem, and hang them upside down to dray for a week or two. Once dried, remove the leaves or flowers from the stem and store in a dry, airtight container. They should last for a year. Dried herbs make excellent teas and food seasoning (see Chapter 3 for instructions).

- **To freeze herbs:** Chop up the clean herbs and place teaspoons full into cells of an ice cube tray. Fill the tray with water and freeze. The benefit of freezing is that herbs retain their just-picked flavor. When needed, just pop out an ice cube and put into a pot or cup like you would fresh herbs.

Chapter 6

Resources

By now, you are equipped with the foundational knowledge of using incorporating herbs into your daily life. Herbalism is an extensive field that requires continuous learning. Here are some of the most authoritative sources that will get you well on your way towards expanding your expertise on the subject.

Encyclopedia of Herbal Medicine: The Definitive Home Reference Guide to 550 Key Herbs with all their Uses as Remedies for Common Ailments
By Andrew Chevallier
(ISBN-10: 0789467836 / ISBN-13: 978-0789467836)

Homegrown Herbs: A Complete Guide to Growing, Using, and Enjoying More than 100 Herbs
By Tammi Hartung
(ISBN-10: 1603427031 / ISBN-13: 978-1603427036)

Growing Herbs at Home: A Guide to Growing Herbs at Home for Beginners
By Charlie Hughes

(ISBN-10: 1517269245 / ISBN-13: 978-1517269241)

The Complete Medicinal Herbal: A Practical Guide to the Healing Properties of Herbs, with More Than 250 Remedies for Common Ailments

By Penelope Ody

(ISBN-10: 156458187X / ISBN-13: 978-1564581877)

Conclusion

Herbalism is practice that is as old as civilization. Long before the advent of modern medicine and chemical engineering that make pharmaceutical development possible, our ancestors had always relied on nature for healing. In fact, without the knowledge of the natural world from the past, there would not have been the foundation which modern medicine was built upon. However, the advancements made in the field of modern medicine are not without their drawbacks to our well-being and the environment.

With that awareness, it is only sensible that we take advantage of what the natural world has to offer, in terms of our overall health and well-being. You now have at your fingertips the knowledge to utilize the gifts of the earth. The rest is all up to you!

www.ingramcontent.com/pod-product-compliance
Lightning Source LLC
Chambersburg PA
CBHW071301280526
45788CB00004B/1807